Fabio Figueiró Tavares

Urinary Antigens in the Diagnosis of CAP in Hospitalized Adults

Fabio Figueiró Tavares

Urinary Antigens in the Diagnosis of CAP in Hospitalized Adults

Etiological Diagnosis in CAP

ScienciaScripts

Imprint
Any brand names and product names mentioned in this book are subject to trademark, brand or patent protection and are trademarks or registered trademarks of their respective holders. The use of brand names, product names, common names, trade names, product descriptions etc. even without a particular marking in this work is in no way to be construed to mean that such names may be regarded as unrestricted in respect of trademark and brand protection legislation and could thus be used by anyone.

Cover image: www.ingimage.com

This book is a translation from the original published under ISBN 978-613-9-62193-4.

Publisher:
Sciencia Scripts
is a trademark of
Dodo Books Indian Ocean Ltd. and OmniScriptum S.R.L publishing group

120 High Road, East Finchley, London, N2 9ED, United Kingdom
Str. Armeneasca 28/1, office 1, Chisinau MD-2012, Republic of Moldova, Europe
Printed at: see last page
ISBN: 978-620-7-71872-6

SUMMARY

DEDICATORY

I dedicate this work to all those who, in some way, believe in human evolution and in the search for knowledge as a tool to bring more comfort and well-being to people.

ACKNOWLEDGMENTS

I'm very grateful to my tutors:

to Dr. José da Silva Moreira, for the attention, cordiality, competence and brilliance with which he plays his role at the head of the Postgraduate Program in Medicine: Pneumology;

to Dr. José Wellington Alves dos Santos, a person of my great esteem and admiration, whose example of discipline and dedication served as a model for my professional training. His tireless struggle, perseverance and commitment to academic activities were my greatest encouragement to enter the master's program.

I would like to thank my parents and my sisters; family who have always been by my side during the most important moments of my life, in which their encouragement, affection and love have laid solid foundations for me to achieve my ideals.

I would like to thank Dr. Alexandre Giacomini and Dr. Gustavo U Rodrigues, people without whom this work would not have been possible, for their valuable logistical support during my years in Porto Alegre.

To Dr. Rubia do Nascimento, a companion of all hours, whose professionalism, tenacity and eagerness for intellectual growth influenced and motivated me to seek out new challenges. Her example and support were essential to the completion of this work.

To Dr. Roseane Marchiori, the shaper of my education, whose knowledge imparted to me during my training as a pulmonologist provided a solid basis for following my professional and academic path.

To Dr. Gustavo Michel for his indispensable support, both in the preparation and progress of this project, which made it possible to carry it out.

To the contracted doctors, resident doctors, monitors, students and staff of the Pneumology Service of the University Hospital of Santa Maria, for their dedication, commitment and the quality of the help provided over the years, which made it possible to complete this work.

SUMMARY

OBJECTIVE: To determine the frequency of community-acquired pneumonia (CAP) caused by *pneumococcus,* using the urinary antigen detection test for *Streptococcus pneumoniae* in hospitalized immunocompetent adults. To evaluate the performance of sputum tests and blood cultures, as well as to describe the clinical, radiological, epidemiological and prognostic aspects associated with CAP.

METHODS: Over a period of 17 months, 30 consecutive patients diagnosed with CAP were prospectively studied.

RESULTS: Seventeen (57%) patients were men, the mean age was 49 years, 14 (48.3%) had comorbidities, 17 (57%) belonged to Fine classes IV and V and 11 (36.7%) patients were admitted to the intensive care unit (ICU). An etiologic agent was identified in 19 of the 30 cases (63%). *Streptococcus pneumoniae* was identified in 14 cases (47%) and accounted for 74% of the etiological diagnoses obtained. The membrane immunochromatographic test (BINAX NOW) identified *S. pneumoniae* in 11 of the 30 cases (36.7%), and was positive in 33% of the cases of unknown etiology using conventional sputum and blood culture methods. The use of antimicrobials prior to hospital admission occurred in 31% of cases and was significantly associated with unknown etiology. Membrane immunochromatographic testing was not affected by the use of antibiotics prior to hospital admission and patients with a positive test had a longer hospital stay.

CONCLUSIONS: In our study, the urinary antigen detection test for *S. pneumoniae* (BINAX NOW) proved to be a useful diagnostic tool in the evaluation of patients with community-acquired pneumonia caused by penumococcus.

INTRODUCTION

Pneumonia is defined by pathologists as an acute, exclusive or predominant inflammation of the lung parenchyma. When of an infectious nature, an inflammatory exudate usually fills the air spaces distal to the terminal bronchioles, consisting of microorganisms, leukocytes, red blood cells and fibrin. In clinical practice, pneumonic syndrome is manifested by acute symptoms (usually cough, expectoration, chest pain and fever). The physical findings on the chest can range from a slight change in the auscultation of the lungs to the presence of percussion tenderness and a tubal murmur, which usually coincide with the type of lesion seen on the chest X-ray.[1,2,3]

Community-acquired pneumonia (CAP) is pneumonia that affects an individual outside of a hospital environment, or occurs within 48 hours of the patient being admitted.[4] CAP is a serious public health problem worldwide, recognized as a potentially fatal disease. Several studies dating back to the pre-antibiotic era reveal an overall mortality from CAP of 1 per 1000 individuals / year, ranging from 20 to 40% among patients affected by this type of pneumonia.[6] At the beginning of the 20th century, *S. pneumoniae* was identified as the causative agent of more than 80% of pneumonia cases, reaching 95% in cases of lobar pneumonia.[5,6]

Streptococcus pneumoniae was isolated simultaneously by Pasteur and Sternberg in 1881. It is a gram-positive, catalase-negative, facultatively anaerobic bacterium that most often grows as a lance-shaped diplococcus,[7] but also as an isolated coccus or in short chains (image 1 and 2)[9,10] . On blood agar, the colonies are alpha-hemolytic, surrounded by a green or brown discoloration of the medium, which is caused by the partial lysis of red blood cells (image 3) .[11]

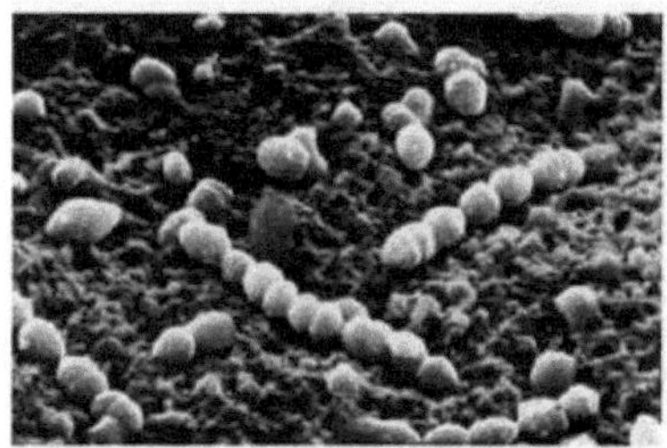

Image 1: *S. pneumoniae* in chains

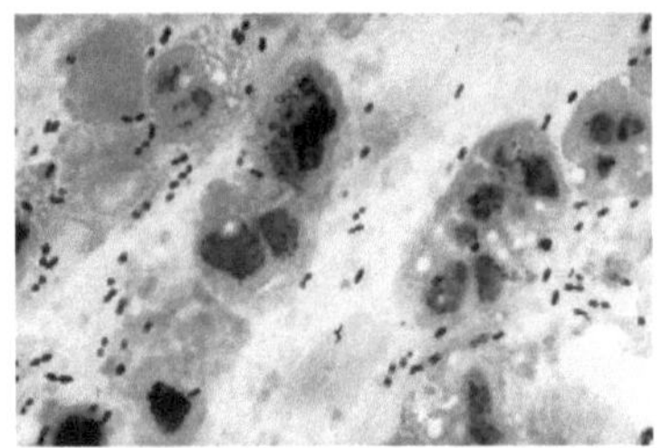

Image 2: *S. pneumoniae* in sputum

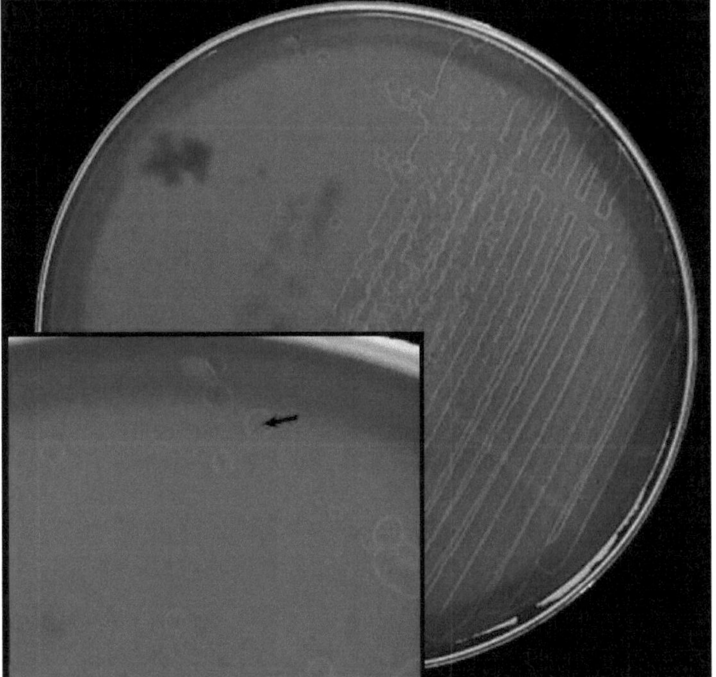

Image 3: Culture plate revealing alpha-hemolysis

The isolated strains are also serotyped on the basis of the capsular polysaccharide that surrounds the cell wall. Ninety different serotypes are known, which are numbered according to the order in which they are identified (American system) or are grouped by antigenic characteristics (Danish system), the latter being the most accepted model. Not all serotypes are able to cause disease; capsular polysaccharide is the major virulence factor, and those strains that produce large amounts of polysaccharide also protect the pathogen by inhibiting the action of phagocytes and complement.[8]

Despite the large number of serotypes, only 10% of the most frequent ones account for 62% of invasive pneumococcal diseases. The distribution of serotypes differs geographically and the predominance of a serotype can change over time. Thus, types 1 and 5 are more common in parts of Europe and in developing countries, but not in the United States.[8]

Streptococcus pneumoniae is transmitted from person to person by droplets of respiratory secretions. It colonizes the upper airways and is part of the normal flora of healthy individuals. Asymptomatic colonization is especially high in children. The rate of nasopharyngeal carriers varies from 5 to 30% in healthy adults and 20 to 50% in children. Pneumonia occurs when microorganisms are carried into the lower airways and overwhelm the host's defenses. The organism causes disease by contiguous dissemination or by hematologic dissemination to distant sites.[8,88]

The current incidence of CAP in adults ranges from 1.6 to 13.4 per 1,000 inhabitants, with hospitalizations ranging from 22% to 54%.[12,13,89] American estimates show that the disease affects 2 to 3 million people every year, resulting in approximately 10 million medical visits, 600,000 hospitalizations and 45,000 deaths.[12,14,15,16] It is the most common cause of death among infectious diseases and the seventh leading cause of death overall.[14] It is estimated that more than 20 billion dollars are spent on treating CAP every year in the United States.[17]

There are few studies on the frequency of CAP in Brazil. It is estimated that there are 2,100,000 cases a year.[2] Data from the Ministry of Health shows that pneumonia is the leading cause of hospitalization, excluding external causes, accounting for 726,366 cases in 2005 (Table 1).[18]

TABLE 1 Hospital morbidity in Brazil (Jan 2005 to Dec 2005)

Illness	Number of Cases
Pneumonia	726.366
Cancer	431.231
Asthma	293.427
STROKE	199.939
COPD	180.101

Diabetes	121.810
IAM	56.345

Source: DATASUS 2006

Currently, the mortality rate varies according to the group studied, corresponding to less than 5% in outpatients, more than 10% in hospitalized patients and on average 36% in those requiring ICU admission.[19,20,21,22,23,90]

Several current studies in various geographical areas of the world point to Streptococcus pneumoniae as the most common pathogen in CAP. Its incidence varies between studies and is much lower than that reported in studies from the pre-antibiotic era (TABLE 2).[24,25,26,27,28,29]

Table 2: Incidence of *S. pneumoniae*

PAiSES	**n**	**% CAP PNEUMOCOCIC**
Taiwan	448	24%
United Kingdom	267	48%
Finland	304	47%
The Netherlands	334	27%
Israel	346	43%
Thailand	147	22%
Japan	232	24%
Argentina	346	24%
Chile	200	40%

In a review of 15 studies of CAP in hospitalized patients published in the United States and Canada, Bartlett and Mundy concluded that over a period of three decades the most frequently identified agent was *S. pneumoniae* (20-60% of all cases). In this review, the etiologic agent remained unknown in 20 to 70% of cases.1,30,31,32,33

Ruiz-Gonzâlez et al, incorporating genetic methods and antigen detection tests in samples obtained through transcutaneous lung puncture, identified a causative agent in 65% of patients with an unknown diagnosis using conventional methods. *S. pneumoniae* was isolated in 33% of these cases, concluding that it is responsible for the vast majority of cases of unknown etiology.[3] 4 Bartlett and Mundy, when analyzing the yield of sputum cultures in patients with bacteremic pneumococcal pneumonia, found a false-negative rate of 50%, which reflects how much the prevalence of *S. pneumoniae* is underestimated and not identified through conventional methods.[35]

The difficulty in identifying *S. pneumoniae* as the causative agent of CAP is influenced by various aspects, such as the difficulty in obtaining good quality sputum, the use of antimicrobial therapy prior to hospitalization and the low yield of blood cultures. In addition, invasive and expensive procedures cannot be used on a daily basis. Therefore, the initial therapeutic decision is often empirical and should be based on preliminary etiological studies and local epidemiological data.[2,21,36,37,38]

Previous antigenic tests, such as latex agglutination or counterimmunoelectrophoresis, including those that detect individual serotypes, have lacked the sensitivity and specificity to gain acceptance as a useful routine technique in clinical practice.[39,91]

A quick and practical test for detecting *S. pneumoniae* capsular antigens in urine (BINAX NOW) has recently been developed. It is capable of detecting 44 different strains, representing the 23 serotypes responsible for more than 90% of infections.[39,40,41]

TIM (BINAX NOW) is a simple, fast, useful method for both outpatients and inpatients. It is non-invasive, offers visually detectable results, long persistence of positivity even after antimicrobial therapy, and is extremely useful in cases not diagnosed by conventional methods. It also has a sensitivity of 78% in non-bacteremic patients and 82-86% in bacteremic patients, with a specificity of > 95%.[41,42,43,44]

OBJECTIVES

a. Main

To determine the frequency of community-acquired pneumonia (CAP) due to *pneumococcus*, using the urinary antigen detection test for *Streptococcus pneumoniae,* in immunocompetent adults admitted to a University Hospital located in the center of the state of Rio Grande do Sul.

b. Secondary

To evaluate the performance of sputum smears and blood cultures in determining the etiologic agent.

Determine the correlation between the Membrane Immunochromatographic Test (MIT) and blood cultures and sputum tests.

Describe the epidemiological, laboratory, radiological and prognostic aspects associated with CAP.

MATERIAL AND METHODS

Patients

Between July 2005 and December 2006, consecutive patients over the age of 14 with a clinical diagnosis of community-acquired pneumonia (CAP) admitted to the University Hospital of Santa Maria, a 350-bed teaching institution that provides tertiary care to an estimated population of 800,000 people in the central region of Rio Grande do Sul, were prospectively studied.

Inclusion criteria

All adult immunocompetent patients admitted with a provisional diagnosis of CAP were included. CAP was defined as the presence of a new pulmonary infiltrate consistent with infection, on a chest radiogram at admission (not pre-existing or justified by any other cause), associated with the acute presentation of any of the major criteria described by Fang et al (axillary temperature > 37.8° C, cough or expectoration), or at least two minor criteria (pleuritic chest pain, dyspnea, leukocyte count > 12.000/mm^3 , altered mental state or lung consolidation on clinical examination).[30]

Exclusion criteria

Patients were excluded if: (a) pneumonia was not the main cause of hospitalization, (b) it was an expected terminal event or (c) it was distal to a bronchial obstruction. Patients with tuberculosis, human immunodeficiency virus (HIV) infection, solid or hematological tumors undergoing chemotherapy, neutropenic (leukocytes < 1,500/mm^3), undergoing chemotherapy with immunosuppressants (cyclosporine, azathioprine) in the six months prior to admission or treatment with doses ≥ 20mg/day of prednisone or its equivalent for at least 30 days in the six months prior to admission were also excluded.

Data collection

Data on the following variables were recorded: age, gender, race, symptoms, physical examination signs, previous antimicrobial therapy for any indication, pneumococcal vaccination, alcohol abuse, smoking, presence of comorbidities and previous history of illnesses.

Risk stratification of patients on hospital admission followed the criteria described by Fine et al.[21]

Microbiological and laboratory analysis

Within 48 hours of hospital admission, blood samples were collected for blood culture (two) and laboratory evaluation: blood count, electrolytes, renal and liver function tests, blood glucose and arterial gasometry. Sputum was collected by spontaneous or induced methods and the sample was considered to be of good quality when it had less than 10 epithelial cells and more than 25 polymorphonuclear leukocytes per small magnification field.[45] In the presence of significant pleural effusion (fluid column > 10 mm on lateral decubitus X-ray), thoracentesis was performed with cytological, biochemical and microbiological analysis of the pleural fluid. All clinical specimens obtained were subjected to direct testing for bacteria (Gram stain), fungi (10% KOH) and acid-fast bacilli (Ziehl-Neelsen stain) and sown on bacteriological (blood agar, chocolate agar, McConkey agar), mycological (Sabouraud agar) and *Mycobacterium tuberculosis (*Lowenstein-Jensen) culture media.

Urine samples were collected, cooled and then warmed to room temperature for the urine antigen detection test. The test consists of an immunochromatographic assay on a nitrocellulose membrane, where rabbit anti-S. *pneumoniae* antibodies and a control anti-species antibody are fixed in separate bands. In addition, there are free rabbit anti-S. *pneumoniae antibodies* and free anti-species antibodies, conjugated to particles that allow visualization. These free complexes are adsorbed onto the nitrocellulose membrane.[46]

The pneumococcal antigen present in the sample reacts with the conjugated anti-S. *pneumoniae* antibody. The resulting antigen-antibody complex is captured by the immobilized anti-S. *pneumoniae antibody*, forming the test band. The immobilized anti-species antibody captures the anti-species conjugate, forming the control band.[46]

To carry out the test, dip the swab into the urine sample and then insert it into the appropriate hole in the book-shaped device (image 4). 3 drops of reagent are applied to the swab and the device is closed. The result is read after 15 minutes in an external window which shows a pink control band and another pink band from the urine sample if the test is positive.[46]

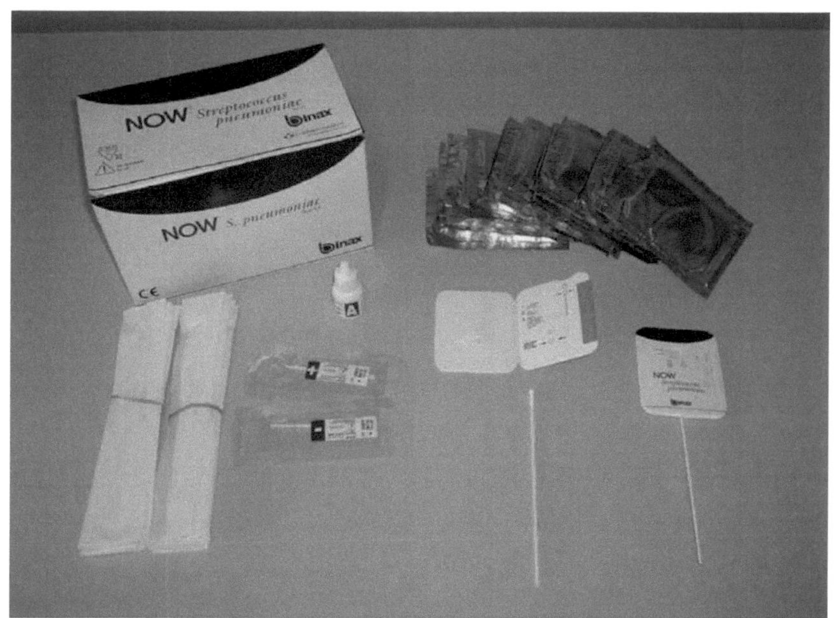

Image 4: BINAX NOW kit for the detection of *S.pneumoniae*

Radiological Analysis

Radiological findings were assessed for the presence of:

- alveolar-ductal consolidation;
- interstitial infiltrate;
- air bronchogram;
- involvement of a single segment (segmental opacity);
- involvement of > 2 segments in a single lobe (lobar opacity);
- involvement of > 2 lobes on a single side (multilobar opacity);
- bilateral involvement;
- presence of pleural effusion;
- presence of cavities.

Criteria for the etiological classification of pneumonia

The identification of the etiological agent was considered a **definite** cause of CAP if there was: [1] isolation in blood culture, pleural fluid culture; **probable** if there was: [1] positive urine antigen test for *Streptococcus pneumoniae,* [2] growth of a predominant bacterial pathogen in sputum culture in combination with Gram stain; and **possible** if there was: [1] gram valid sputum sample with a predominance of gram-positive diplococci, gram-positive cocci in clusters, gram-negative cocobacilli, [2] isolation of a pathogen in the sputum culture in the absence of compatible direct examination.[3]

The etiology of CAP was considered **mixed** when more than one microorganism was found according to the above criteria.

Aspiration pneumonia was considered when no microbiological diagnosis was obtained in a patient with a condition predisposing to aspiration (swallowing disorders or altered consciousness), associated with a new infiltrate in a pending lung segment.[33]

Unknown etiology was defined as failure to obtain an etiological diagnosis.

Statistical analysis

The results are presented as mean and standard deviation. Continuous variables were compared using the Student's t-test or Mann-Whitney test when appropriate, and categorical variables were compared using the Chi-square test. A significance level of 5.0% ($p < 0.05$) was adopted.

The data was analyzed and processed using SPSS® version 11.0 for Windows®.

Ethical issues

This project was approved by the Ethics Committee of the University Hospital of Santa Catarina.

Maria.

RESULTS

Patients' general characteristics

Three patients were excluded from the study, 1 of whom had AIDS, 1 chronic myelocytic leukemia, and 1 whose chest X-ray did not confirm the presence of pneumonia.

A total of 30 patients hospitalized for CAP met the inclusion criteria. The clinical and epidemiological characteristics of this group are described in Tables 3 and 4. Seventeen patients (57%) were men, twenty-five (83%) were white. The age of the 30 patients ranged from 20 to 80 years (49 ± 20.4 years). Thirteen patients (49%) were smokers and two (7%) were alcoholics. Fourteen (48%) had comorbidities, the most frequently observed of which were COPD (24%), diabetes mellitus (17%) and heart disease (10%).

None of the patients had been previously vaccinated against Pneumococcus. Nine of the thirty patients (31%) had used antimicrobial therapy prior to hospital admission. The average time between the onset of symptoms and hospitalization was eight days (±8). The most frequent symptoms were: cough (97%), fever (86%), dyspnea (83%), chest pain (72%) and expectoration (63%). Twenty-five (89%) had altered pulmonary auscultation. Mental confusion was present in ten of the thirty patients (36%). Seventeen (57%) patients belonged to Fine classes IV and V, and eleven (37%) were admitted to the ICU.

The hospital stay was 12 ± 10 days. Eleven of the thirty patients (37%) presented complications during their evolution, such as heart failure, myocardial ischemia, septic shock, acute renal failure, respiratory failure and pleural empyema. Four patients (13%) died.

TABLE 3 - Clinical characteristics of Iiospitalized patients (n=30)

CLINICAL CHARACTERISTICS	n (%)
Coughing	28 (96,6%)
Expectoration	19 (63,3%)
Dyspnea	24 (82,8%)
Chest pain	21 (72,4%)
Altered consciousness	10 (35,7%)

Upper airway symptoms	8 (27,6%)
Systemic symptoms	26 (89,7%)
Fever	25 (86,2%)
Arthralgia	4 (13,8%)
Anorexia	12 (41,4%)
Sweating	12 (41,4%)
Myalgia	7 (24,1%)
Lymphadenopathy	0 (0%)
Altered pulmonary auscultation	25 (89,3%)

TABLE 4 Epidemiological characteristics of hospitalized patients (n=30)

CHARACTERISTICS	n (%)
Male	17 (56,7%)
Age (years)	49+20,4(20-80)*
White color	25 (83,3%)
Black Brown Smoking Alcoholism	2 (6,7%)
	3 (10,0%)
	13 (44,8%)
	2 (6,9%)
Comorbidities	14 (48,3%)
COPD	7 (24,1%)
Heart disease	3 (10,3%)
Neoplasm	0 (0%)
Diabetes mellitus	5 (17,2%)
Neurological disease	2 (6,9%)

Liver disease	2 (6,9%)
Kidney disease	2 (6,9%)
Pneumococcal vaccination Hospital complications Prior antimicrobial use ICU admission	0 (0%) 11 (36,7%) 9 (31%) 11 (36,7%)
Hospital stay	
Time elapsed between onset of symptoms and hospitalization	13 + 10 days (2-49)*
Duration of treatment	8 + 8 days (1-32)*
Time between onset of symptoms and urine collection	12 + 6 days (1-32)* 10 + 8 days (1-32)*
Mortality	4 (13,0%)

* Arithmetic mean ± standard deviation (range).

Radiological picture

The vast majority (89.0%) had a chest radiogram with an alveolar-ductal pattern, 44.8% with bilateral distribution and 31.0% with lobar distribution. Parapneumonic pleural effusion was seen in 8 cases (27.6%), but in only 3 was it significant, requiring diagnostic thoracentesis. Other characteristics are summarized in Table 5.

TABLE 5 Radiological characteristics (n=30).

CHANGES	TOTAL	%
Alveolar-ductal consolidation	26	89,7
Air bronchogram	7	24,1
Interstitial infiltrate	2	6,9

Involvement of a	Single segment	
(segmental opacity)	4	13,8
Involvement of >2 segments in a single case		
lobe (lobar opacity)	9	31,0
Involvement of >2 lobes	on one side only	
(multilobar opacity)	2	6,9
Bilateral involvement	13	44,8
Presence of pleural effusion	8	26,6
Presence of cavities	1	3,4

Diagnostic Methods

The diagnostic methods used and the proportion of positive cases for each method are summarized in tables 6, 7 and 8.

Sputum was obtained from 19 of the 30 patients (63.3%). Of these, only 14 (46.7%) met the Murray-Washington acceptance criteria.[45] Among these 14 valid samples, numerous gram-positive cocci in pairs or chains were present in eight cases (57.1% of the valid samples).

The sputum cultures were positive in only six samples, 1 for *Staphylococcus aureus*, 1 *Streptococcus sp* 1 *Enterococcus fecalis* and 3 *Streptococcus pneumoniae*. There was agreement between the growth of a predominant pathogen in the sputum culture and what was observed on Gram stain in all six (43% of the valid samples).

Blood cultures were taken from 23 of the 30 patients (76.7%). Of these, 4 (17.3%) were positive, 1 for *Escherichia coli,* 1 for *Staphylococcus aureus*, 1 for *Streptococcus viridans* and 1 for *Streptococcus pneumoniae.*

Three patients presented with significant parapneumonic pleural effusion during the course of treatment and required thoracentesis. Pleural fluid culture was negative in all three.

The membrane immunochromatographic test (MIT) was carried out on the urine of all 30 patients, and was positive in 11 cases (36.7%). Of these cases, seven produced adequate sputum samples, in which the presence of gram-positive cocci arranged in pairs was observed in five (71.4% of valid samples). In only 3 of the 11 cases of positive TIM, the sputum culture showed growth of *Streptococcus pneumoniae* in agreement with the gram stain, and only 1 produced a positive blood culture for Pneumococcus.

TIM was also carried out on the pleural fluid of two patients who had complicated parapneumonic pleural effusions, both of whom tested positive. These patients had already tested positive in the urine sample.

TABLE 6 - Direct examination of sputum in valid samples (n=14).

	№ CASES	(%)
Sputum with a predominance of gram-positive cocci positive in pairs or chains	8	57%
Sputum with a predominance of others microorganisms	4	29%
Germ-free sputum	2	14%

TABLE 7 - Cultural examination of sputum in valid samples (n=14).

	№ CASES	(%)
Positive culture for *S. pneumoniae*	3	21%
Positive culture for others microorganisms	3	21%
Negative sputum culture	8	58%

TABLE 8. Other diagnostic methods.

METHODS	CASES REALIZED (n)	CASES POSITIVE (n)	POSITIVITY (%)
Blood cultures	23	4	17,3
Pleural fluid culture	3	0	0,0
TIM	30	11	36,7

Etiological diagnosis

Nineteen patients had an etiological agent identified (63%). The diagnosis was definitive in 4 cases, probable in 12, and possible in 3. There was 1 case of mixed etiology. It was not possible to determine a causal agent of CAP in 11 patients (37%), who were labeled as cases of unknown etiology (table 9).

The etiological diagnosis of CAP due to *Streptococcus pneumoniae* occurred in 13 cases (43%), and represented 68% of the etiological diagnoses obtained. Eleven patients had positive TIM. Eight patients had a predominance of gram-positive cocci in pairs or chains in their sputum, and in three of these there was agreement between the culture and the direct examination. There was one case of bacteremia. Two patients had complicated parapneumonic effusions in this group, which required closed pleural drainage.

Etiological diagnosis of pneumonia, in which other pathogens were found

involved, was carried out on 5 patients. In this group, 2 patients were diagnosed with

definitive and 3 probable, according to the agreement between the results of the direct examination of the sputum with its culture and blood cultures.

There was one case of mixed etiology. In this case, *S. aureus* was isolated in a blood culture associated with positive TIM.

TABLE 9 - Etiology of CAP in hospitalized patients (n=30).

ETIOLOGY	DEFINITIVE	PROBABLE	POSSIBLE	TOTAL	%
S. pneumoniae	1	10	3	13	43
Other pathogens	2	3	0	5	17
Mixed etiology	1	1	-	1	3
Etiology unknown	-	-	-	11	37

Prognostic factors

The results of the prognostic factors and risk stratification of the patients are summarized in Tables 10 and 11. A total of 17 patients (57%) had a Fine score > IV. There was a significant association between a Fine score > 122 and ICU admission ($p = 0.03$).

Eleven patients (36.7%) were admitted to the ICU. Of these, 8 (73%) had a Fine score > IV, and seven (64%) had comorbidities. Nine (82%) had a respiratory rate > 30 and a heart rate > 125; eight (73%) had a PaO2 < 60. SBP < 90 occurred in 8 patients (27.6%) and was significantly associated with ICU admission (p=0.035).

The mortality rate was 13%.

TABLE 10. Prognostic factors in adults hospitalized for CAP (n=30).

PROGNOSTIC FACTORS	PATIENTS	%
Age ≥ 65 years	8	27
Male	17	56,7
Comorbidities	14	48,3
Altered mental state	10	35,7
Systemic BP < 90mmHg	8	27,6
Respiratory rate ≥ 30 /min	16	55,2
Heart rate ≥ 125 /min	17	58,6
Temperature < 35 or > 40 C°	5	17,2
Serum urea >30 mg/dl	12	41,4
Serum sodium < 130 mEq/l	2	6,9
Hematocrit < 30%	2	6,9
Glucose > 250mg%	1	3,4
Arterial pH < 7.35	2	6,9
PaO2 < 60mmHg or O2 sat < 90%	11	37,9
Pleural effusion	8	27,6
ICU admission	11	36,7
Fine index > IV	17	57
Deaths	4	13,0

TABLE 11. Risk stratification of patients hospitalized for CAP (n=30).

FINE CLASS	**PATIENTS**	**%**
FINE I	2	6,7
FINE II	3	10,0
FINE III	8	26,7
FINE IV	14	46,7
FINE V	3	10,0
Fine Index ≥ IV	17	57,0

DISCUSSION

The microbiological diagnosis of community-acquired pneumonia (CAP) has been obtained in 42% to 88% of cases, with considerable differences between studies in the frequency of causative agents, due to factors that include: seasonal, geographical, epidemiological and methodological variations, as well as admission criteria for hospitalized patients and, above all, the diagnostic methods used.[24,30,47,48,49,50]

Etiology studies have failed to find a causative agent for pneumonia in half of the cases. One hypothesis is that many of these cases are due to *S. pneumoniae*, which appears to be the most important agent responsible for CAP that is not identified by conventional methods.[34,40]

In the present series - taking into account the use of all the methods employed - the etiology of pneumonia was clarified in 19 of the 30 cases (63%) and, as in most studies, *S. pneumoniae* was the main agent isolated (in 14 cases, 47%), which represented 74% of the cases clarified.[51,52,53] If we only consider conventional diagnostic methods, the etiology would be clarified in only 14 cases (47%) - 4 with a definitive diagnosis, 5 with a suggestive diagnosis and 5 cases of possible etiology. The etiology would then be unknown in 53% of cases. Using TIM, it was possible to identify 31% of the cases that would have had an unknown etiology if only conventional methods had been used; in these cases, the probable etiology was *S. pneumoniae.* These data are in line with the literature, which estimates that *S. pneumoniae is* responsible for approximately 1/3 of cases with unknown etiology.27,41,42,54,55

Most studies on the etiology of CAP recognize that in 3 to 14% of patients, two or more pathogens can be identified as the cause of the infection.[56] One study, however, showed that 35% of pneumococcal infections were mixed, with the most frequently found agents being *C. pneumoniae, M. pneumoniae* and viruses.[25] There was only 1 case of mixed etiology in the present series. This underestimated frequency probably occurred because serological tests for atypical germs and viral agents were not carried out.

Conventional tests for the etiological investigation of pneumonia are imperfect: the value of sputum cultures is uncertain, since their positivity can be the result of colonization, blood cultures are positive in an infinite number of cases and lack sensitivity and, although serological analyses are reliable, they do not provide results in sufficient time to be clinically useful for therapy.[34,40]

According to Fang et al[30] and Bohte et al[47] , direct sputum examination complemented by culture, when collected, processed and interpreted properly, is a very important method for quickly identifying the etiological agent, guiding initial therapy and allowing knowledge of the sensitivity profile of microorganisms to antimicrobials.

Bartlett and Mundy, in a review of 15 studies in North America, concluded that approximately 10-30% of patients with CAP do not expectorate, and that good quality sputum is not obtained in more than 50% of them. Around 15-30% have received antibiotics prior to investigation, and 30-65% of sputum cultures yield negative results.[35]

When efforts are made to collect sputum, the results are high. Gecker et al[57] obtained a sample in 96% of patients by combining nebulization with saline solution and postural drainage when necessary. In contrast, Marrie et al[58] obtained success in only 36%.[59]

The sensitivity of sputum cultures is low. A review of 11 studies carried out in 1999 by Skerrett et al[60] , found diagnostic yields ranging from 20-79%. Sensitivity and specificity were reduced by contamination with colonizing flora from the upper respiratory tract and previous antibiotic therapy.[59] Several more current studies reveal a frequency of previous antibiotic use ranging from 23 - 63.8%, which certainly contributes to a reduction of up to 4 times the etiological diagnostic yield of CAP. 26,61,62,63,64

These facts together explain the discrepancy between studies that reveal sensitivities ranging from 20-69% for gram and 29-94% for culture.[24,62]

In this study, sputum samples were obtained from 19 patients (63.3%), of which 14 (47%) met the Murray-Washington acceptance criteria. Of these, 12 showed a predominance of some microorganism, and in 6 (43% of the valid samples) there was growth of a predominant pathogen in the culture in combination with gram stain, which corresponds to 20% of all 30 patients. This low yield can be attributed to the difficulty in obtaining a sputum sample and the high rate of antibiotic therapy prior to hospitalization, present in 31% of cases.

Rosón et al[65] compared the sensitivity of direct sputum examination and the membrane immunochromatographic test (TIM) for diagnosing pneumococcal CAP in bacteremic patients. TIM showed a sensitivity of 92% and gram 25%. Rosón concluded that TIM proved to be sensitive and highly specific, being especially useful in cases where sputum is inconclusive. In the present study, TIM detected 11 out of 14 cases of pneumococcal CAP, and direct sputum examination 8 cases. Of the 11 patients with a positive TIM, 7 produced a valid sputum sample, five of which showed gram-positive cocci in pairs or short chains on direct examination (71.4% of the valid samples).

In most epidemiological studies of CAP, blood culture positivity ranges from 4% to 18%, and is higher in severe pneumonia.[31,33,66,67,68,92,93] Of the 30 patients in this study, blood culture samples were collected from 23, and it was possible to establish the diagnosis in 17.3% of the specimens collected (25% *S. pneumoniae, 25% S. aureus, 25% E. coli* and 25% *S. viridans*).

As well as being an important diagnostic method, blood cultures allow antibiograms to be drawn up which help in the choice of therapy and allow continuous monitoring of the resistance rates of *S. pneumoniae*. Meta-analysis studies show that the mortality rate for penicillin-resistant pneumococci is 30% higher than for susceptible strains.69

The presence of bacteremia is associated with a worse prognosis, with approximately 25% of pneumococcal CAPs having bacteremia, constituting a group with a higher mortality rate. Probably due to the small sample size, this relationship could not be ascertained in this study.[29,70,71,72,73]

There is controversy about the routine use of blood cultures in CAP. Some authors raise the issue of cost-benefit and the low yield of blood cultures. In addition, there is evidence that changing therapy based on blood culture results does not seem to change mortality. The results of blood cultures are generally used infrequently to change therapy, especially when the pathogens isolated are sensitive to antibiotics with a lower spectrum of action. Other facts also contribute to this approach: the contamination rate of blood cultures is as high as 5%, and these false-positive results increase the length of hospitalization; the yield of blood cultures is affected by the previous use of antibiotics; and patients with pneumococcal bacteremia do not require a longer course of antibiotic therapy than non-bacteremic patients.[67,74]

In our study, TIM was positive in the case of *S. pneumoniae* bacteremia. Previous studies have shown a sensitivity of 70.4% to 89.7% and specificity of 89.7% to 97% for TIM when tested against blood cultures, which are considered the gold standard. Although new diagnostic tests are compared with blood cultures, bacteremia is documented in only 20-30% of cases of pneumococcal pneumonia.[39,40,41,42]

Parapneumonic effusions are found in 20 to 60% of patients with community-acquired pneumonia.[35] Most evolve well with antibiotic treatment. It is estimated that 10% of cases complicate and require pleural drainage.[35] In this study, eight of the thirty patients (26.6%) developed parapneumonic pleural effusion. Of these, three (10%) had complicated effusions and required closed drainage. Microbiological analysis was negative in all three, and they were *already* receiving intravenous antibiotic therapy. TIM was carried out on the pleural fluid of two of them, and was positive in both. These two patients had already had a positive urine TIM result.

The immunochromatographic test for the detection of pneumococcal antigens was developed for use on urine or cerebrospinal fluid. There are no studies validating its usefulness in other types of samples such as plasma and body fluids. Its use as a tool for detecting complicated parapneumonic pleural effusion remains to be proven by subsequent studies.

As already discussed, the use of antibiotics prior to a more specific investigation into the etiology of CAP is associated with a reduction in the sensitivity of conventional microbiological isolation methods, which was also observed in this study. In patients who received antibiotics before hospitalization, there was a significant reduction in the performance of conventional diagnostic methods in finding the etiology of pneumonia compared to those without antibiotics: no cases (0.0%) in 9, compared to nine (45%) in 21 respectively ($p=0.047$). On the other hand, TIM was able to detect the presence of *Streptococcus pneumoniae* in 33% of patients who had received antibiotic therapy prior to hospitalization and in 38% of those who had not (non-significant difference), agreeing with the fact that the diagnostic performance of this test is independent of previous antibiotic therapy.

Considering the cost, simplicity, speed and rate of detection of additional cases, the routine concentration of urine samples for TIM is not justified. The time taken to concentrate urine by ultrafiltration varies from 1 to 4 hours, depending on the characteristics of each specimen. Although urine concentration yielded a 1.4x increase in sensitivity by Marcos et al[75] , this yield was not reproduced by the study by Murdoch et al[40] , and was associated with a lower specificity by Gutierrez et al.[42]

In this study, the urine samples were not concentrated and there was no differentiation between the color intensity of the result lines. Stralin et al[76] reported that the staining of the lines changed from weak to strong intensity after the urine samples were centrifuged. There have also been reports of weak lines in patients with positive blood cultures for *S. pneumoniae*. Dominguez et al[44] considered weak lines to be negative after two patients with false-positive results showed similar lines. These two patients had CAP due to *L. pneumophila and B. fragilis*, but the possibility of a mixed etiology cannot be ruled out.

False-positive TIM results are common in children who are asymptomatic carriers of *S. pneumoniae*, and this decreases with age. The highest rate is found in children under 3 years old (21%), reducing to 11% in those over 3 years old. False-positive results can also occur as a cross-reaction with other *Streptococcus* species such as *S. mitis* and *S. oralis*. However, these pathogens are not associated with CAP.[43]

The radiological analysis of this study revealed that the vast majority (89%) of the patients had an alveolar-ductal pattern on the chest X-ray, with bilateral distribution in 44.8% and lobar distribution in 31%. Air bronchograms were seen in 24.1% of the tests, eight (27.6%) had pleural effusion and only one had a cavity, in which *S. aureus was found in* the blood culture. In general, however, the radiographic findings could not be specifically associated with the type of germ found or with reactivity to TIM.

It should be remembered that community-acquired pneumonia in immunocompetent and previously healthy individuals most often presents radiologically in the form of alveolar-ductal consolidation (pneumococcus, legionella) or with a pattern of interstitial bronchopneumonia (mycoplasma, virus), which in its evolution often also ends up showing areas of consolidation. Macfarlane et al[77] showed that inter-observer reproducibility for distinguishing alveolar from interstitial infiltrates, and lobar from bronchopneumonia, is poor, which implies that it is of little use in predicting the etiology of CAP. Tew et al[78] studied the accuracy of radiological diagnosis for bacterial and non-bacterial pneumonia. The diagnosis was accurate in 16 cases (67%) of bacterial pneumonia and 9 cases (65%) of viral pneumonia.

Ponka and Sarna[79] retrospectively studied 150 patients with PNM caused by viruses,

Mycoplasma and bacteremic pneumonia caused by pneumococcus. They classified the radiological findings as lobar, bronchopneumonic and interstitial. When the presence of these findings was compared between the 3 groups, there was no statistically significant difference. Macfarlane et al[77] reviewed 196 chest X-rays of adults with CAP. They compared 49 cases of pneumonia due to *Legionella sp* with 91 due to pneumococcus, 46 *Mycoplasma pneumoniae and* 10 *Chlamydia psittaci.* The radiological pattern at admission was not useful in differentiating types of pneumonia.

Thus, the results of this study are in line with the current literature, in which there is a consensus that the chest X-ray has a low performance in differentiating the etiological agents that cause CAP.[80,94] It is the characteristics of the patient and their immune status that determine the clinical and radiological picture, much more than the causative agent.[95]

Hospitalization occurs in 20-50% of CAP cases.[25,65,96,97,98] Risk stratification using the pneumonia severity index (PSI) described by Fine et al[21] , reduces the proportion of low-risk patients admitted to hospital without affecting short-term mortality or subsequent hospitalization.[99,100,101] In this series there were five admissions of low-risk patients, Fine class I and II.

There are additional factors that must be taken into account when deciding whether to admit a patient to hospital: important comorbidities not included in the risk stratification schemes (HIV, severe neuromuscular disease, immunosuppression, COPD exacerbation, asthma, CHF, arrhythmia, AMI, digestive hemorrhage, TIA, severe anemia, large pleural effusions, abdominal distension with suspected infectious focus), previous failure of outpatient therapy, social factors (family and financial structure, alcohol and drug abuse), oral intolerance (vomiting), non-compliance with treatment (psychiatric illness), suppurative or metastatic complications such as: empyema, lung abscess, endocarditis, meningitis, osteomyelitis.[21,81,102]

ATS, IDSA and the American College of Emergency Physicians all support the idea that risk stratification schemes cannot replace clinical judgment in indicating hospitalization.[19,36,82] The low-risk patients in this series had at least one of the factors described above, justifying their hospitalization.

There was a significant difference in the length of hospital stay between patients with positive and negative TIM (13 days vs 7 days; $p = 0.022$).The number of days needed for infectious parameters to reach stability depends on comorbidities, characteristics of the CAP, ATB treatment used, complications and the need for ICU admission. Pneumococcus is the most common agent and tends to be associated with more severe disease than several other pathogens.[17,83,103]

The mortality rate from CAP found in the literature is variable, remaining at around 13%,[24,84] and reaching 20-50% in the 10-30% of hospitalized patients who require ICU admission.[85,86] In the present study, the death rate was 13.0%, with no significant difference in mortality between pneumococcal pneumonia and other pneumonia, and no relationship with TIM positivity.

TIM can increase the yield of pathogen identification, and a positive test allows the administration of more targeted therapy against S. pneumoniae. It is especially useful in patients with prior antibiotic therapy and in geographical areas where treatment is complicated by the increase in the number of strains with resistance to penicillin and third-generation cephalosporins.

Some studies have shown that adherence to empirical therapeutic guidelines reduces the need for hospitalization, length of hospital stay, duration of symptoms, length of intravenous treatment, risk of complications and mortality.[19,36,87,104,105,106,107]

The importance of disseminating a therapeutic guide in our country should be emphasized, taking into account the epidemiological information and clinical studies carried out in our country. In this way, empirical treatment should be based on the results of microbiological studies carried out in different geographical areas of the country, associated with local bacterial resistance models.[17,86]

CONCLUSIONS

Using the Membrane Immunochromatographic Test to detect urinary antigen in patients admitted to the University Hospital of Santa Maria (RS) with community-acquired pneumonia (CAP), it was observed that:

1. *S. pneumoniae* was the germ most frequently identified as the cause of CAP, occurring in 36.7% of cases;

2. *S. pneumoniae* was responsible for 33% of pneumonia cases whose cause was unknown using conventional diagnostic methods;

3. TIM sensitivity was not affected by the use of antibiotics prior to hospitalization;

It was also found that:

4. The growth of a predominant pathogen in the sputum culture combined with gram staining and blood culture showed a low yield in the identification of pneumococcus as the etiologic agent of CAP in the sample studied;

5. The direct examination of gram-stained sputum, when well collected, with the presence of gram-positive cocci in pairs or in short chains, proved to be compatible with the probable diagnosis of CAP by *S. pneumoniae* established through the TIM;

6. The clinical and radiological characteristics were neither sensitive nor specific in differentiating pneumonia caused by *S. pneumoniae* from other CAPs;

7. CAP caused by *S. pneumoniae* was associated with a longer hospital stay;

8. Systolic blood pressure lower than 90 mmHg and a FINE score higher than 122 were variables significantly associated with ICU admission;

9. The other epidemiological, laboratory and radiological aspects were similar to those already described in the literature.

BIBLIOGRAPHICAL REFERENCES

1. Marrie T. Community acquired pneumonia. Clin Infect Dis 1994; 18: 501-513.

2. Brazilian Society of Pneumology and Phthisiology. Brazilian Consensus on Pneumonia in Immunocompetent Adults. JPneumol 2001; 27 (Suppl 1): S1-S40.

3. Marrie TJ, Campbell GD, Walker DH, Low DE. Pneumonia. In Harrison's principles of Internal Medicine 16th part 9; 1528-1541.

4. Brazilian Society of Pneumology and Phthisiology. Guideline for Community-Acquired Pneumonia (CAP) in Immunocompetent Adults. J Brasileiro de Pneumologia 2004; 30 (Supl 4): S1-S24.

5. Heffron R. Pneumonia, with special reference to pneumococcal lobar pneumonia. Cambridge, Mass.: Harvard University Press, 1979; 302-8.

6. Bullowa JGM. The reliability of sputum typing and its relation to serum therapy. JAMA 1935; 105: 1512-8.

7. Bauer T, Ewig S, Marcos MA, Werninghaus GS, Torres A. *Streptococcus pneumoniae* in community-acquired pneumonia: how important is drug resistance? Med Clin N Am 2001; 85: 1367-79.

8. Pappas AEB, Margolis MB, Center KJ, Isaacman DJ. *Streptococcus pneumoniae*: description of the pathogen, disease, epidemiology, treatment, and prevention. Pharmacotherapy 2005; 25 (9): 1193-1212.

9. National Physician Chamber Rhineland-Palatinate homepage. Available at http://www.laek-rlp.de. Accessed November 10, 2006.

10. Loyola University Chicago Stritch School of Medicine homepage - Medical education pages. Available at http://www.luc.edu. Accessed on November 10, 2006.

11. Universityof Florida homepage - College of Medicine. Available at http://www.ufl.com. Accessed on November 10, 2006.

12. Almirall J, Bolibar I, Toran P, Pera G, Boquet X, Balanzó X, et al. Contribution of C-Reactive Protein to the Diagnosis and Assessment of Severity of Community-Acquired Pneumonia. Chest 2004; 125: 1335-1342.

13. Working Group of the Latin American Thoracic Association (ALAT). ALAT recommendations on community-acquired pneumonia. Arch Bronconeumol 2001; 37: 340348.

14. Majumdar SR, McAlister FA, Eurich DT, Padwal RS, Marie TJ. Statins and outcomes in patients admitted to hospital with community-acquired pneumonia: population based prospective cohort study. BMJ October 2006; 333:999.

15. Ramsdell J, Narsavage GL, Fink JB. Management of Community-Acquired Pneumonia in the Home: an American college of chest physicians clinical position statement. Chest 2005; 127: 1752-63.

16. Jackson ML, Neuzil KM, Thompson WW, Shay DK, Yu O, Hanson CA, Jackson LA. The Burden of Community-Acquired Pneumonia in Seniors: Results of a Population-Based Study. Clin Infect Dis 2004; 39: 1642-50.

17. File TMJr, Garau J, Blasi F, Chidiac C, Klugman K, Lode H, et al. Guidelines for Empiric Antimicrobial Prescribing in Community-Acquired Pneumonia. Chest 2004; 125: 18881901.

18. Brazil. Ministry of Health. Health Information. Available at http://www.datasus.gov.br. Accessed on: November 20, 2006.

19. Niederman MS, Mandell LA, Anzueto A, Bass JB, Broughton WA, Campbell GD, et al. American Thoracic Society. Guidelines for the management of adults with community-acquired pneumonia. Am J Respir Crit Care Med 2001; 163: 1730-54.

20. Oosterheert JJ, Bonten MJ, Hak E, Schneider MM, Hoepelman AI. Severe community-acquired pneumonia: what's in a name? Curr Opin Infect Dis 2003; 16: 153-9.

21. Fine MJ, Auble TE, Yealy DM, Hanusa BH, Weissfeld LA, Singer DE, et al. A prediction rule to identify low risk patients with community-acquired pneumonia. N Engl J

Med 1997;

336: 243-50.

22. Niederman MS, McCombs JS, Unger NA, et al. The costs of treating community-acquired pneumonia. Clin Ther 1998; 20: 820-837.

23. Medicare and medicaid statistical supplement, 1995. U.S. Department of Health and Human Services, Health Care Financing Administration. Health Care Financ Rev Stat Suppl 1995 (september); 1-388.

24. Luna CM, Famiglietti A, Absi R, Videla AJ, Nogueira FJ, Fuenzalida AD, et al. Community-acquired pneumonia. Etiology, epidemiology, and outcome at a teaching hospital in Argentina. Chest 2000; 118: 1344-54.

25. Jokinen C, Heiskanen L, Juvonen H, Kallinen S, Kleemola M, Koskela M, et al. Microbial Etiology of Community-Acquired Pneumonia in the Adult Population of 4 Municipalities in Eastern Finland. Clin Infect Dis 2001; 32: 1141-54.

26. Saito A, Kohno S, Matsushima T, Watanabe A, Oizumi K, et al. Prospective multicenter study of causative organisms of community-acquired pneumonia in adults in Japan. J Infect Chemother 2006; 12: 63-69.

27. Lauderdale T, Chang F, Ben R, Yin H, et al. Etiology of community acquired pneumonia among adult patients requiring hospitalization in Taiwan. J Respir Med 2005; 99: 10791086.

28. Wattanathum A, Chaoprasong C, Nunthapisud P, Chantaratchada S, Limpairojn N, et al. Community-acquired pneumonia in southwest asia: the microbial differences between ambulatory and hospitalized patients. Chest 2003; 123: 1512-1519.

29. Riquelme RO, Riquelme MO, Rioseco MLZ, Gómez VM, Gil RD, Torres AM. Etiology and prognostic factors of community-acquired pneumonia in hospitalized adults, Puerto Montt, Chile. Ver Méd Chile 2006; 134: 597-605.

30. Fang GD, Fine M, Orloff J, Arisumi D, Yu VL, Kapoor W, et al. New and emerging etiologies for community-acquired pneumonia with implications for therapy. A prospective

multicenter study of 359 cases. Medicine (Baltimore) 1990; 69: 307-16.

31. Marrie TJ, Durant H, Yates L. Community-acquired pneumonia requiring hospitalization: 5-year prospective study. Rev Infect Dis 1989; 11: 586-99.

32. Torres A, Serra-Battles J, Ferrer A. et al. Severe community-acquired pneumonia. Am Rev Resp Dis 1991; 144: 312-318.

33. Mundy LM, Auwaerter PG, Oldach D, Warner ML, Burton A, Vance E, et al. Community- acquired pneumonia: impact of immune status. Am J Respir Crit Care Med 1995; 152: 1309-15.

34. Ruiz-Gonzàlez A, Falguera M, Nogués A, Rubio-Caballero M. Is *Streptococcus pneumoniae* the leading cause of pneumonia of unknown etiology? A microbiologic study of lung aspirates in consecutive patients with community-acquired pneumonia. Am J Med 1999; 106: 385-90.

35. Bartlett JG, Mundy LM. Community-acquired pnemonia. N Engl J Med 1995; 33: 1618-1624.

36. Bartlett JG, Dowell SF, Mandell LA, File TM Jr, Musher DM, Fine MJ. Practice guidelines for the management of community-acquired pneumonia in adults. Infectious Diseases Society of America. Clin Infect Dis 2000; 31: 347-82.

37. Niederman MS, Bass JB Jr, Campbell GD, Fein AM, Grossman RF, Mandell LA, et al. Guidelines for the initial management of adults with community-acquired pneumonia: diagnosis, assessment of severity, and initial antimicrobial therapy. American Thoracic Society. Medical Section of the American Lung Association. Am Rev Respir Dis 1993; 148: 1418-26.

38. Karalus NC, Cunsons RT, Leng RA, et al. Community-acquired pneumonia. An etiology and prognostic index evaluation. Thorax 1991; 46: 413-418.

39. Smith MD, Derrington P, Evans R, Creek M, Morris R, Dance DAB, Cartwright K. Rapid diagnosis of bacteremic pneumococcal infections in adults by using the Binax NOW *Streptococcus pneumoniae* urinary antigen test: a prospective, controlled clinical evaluation.

J Clin Microbiol 2003; 41: 2810-2813.

40. Murdoch DR, Laing RTR, Mills GD, Karalus NC, Town GI, Mirrett S, Reller LB. Evaluation of a rapid immunochromatographic test for detection of Streptococcus pneumoniae antigen in urine samples from adults with community-acquired pneumonia. J Clin Microbiol 2001; 39: 3495-98.

41. Ishida T, Hashimoto T, Arita M, Tojo Y, Tachibana H, Jinnai M. A 3-year Prospective Study for a Urinary Antigen-Detection Test for *Streptococcus pneumoniae* in Community-Acquired Pneumonia: utility and clinical impact on the reported etiology. J Infect Chemother 2004; 10: 359-363.

42. Gutierrez F, Masia M, Rodriguez JC, Ayelo A, Soldan B, Cebrian L, et al. Evaluation of the immunochromatographic Binax NOW assay for detection of *Streptococcus pneumoniae* urinary antigen in a prospective study of community-acquired pneumonia in Spain. Clin Infect Dis 2003; 36: 286-92.

43. Hamer DH, Egas J, Estrella B, MacLeod WB, Grifffths JK, Sempertegui F. Assessment of the Binax NOW *Streptococcus pneumoniae* antigen test in children with nasopharyngeal pneumococcal carriage. Clin Infect Dis 2002; 34: 1025-8.

44. Dominguez J, Gali N, Blanco S, Pedroso P, Prat C, Matas L, Ausina V. Detection of *Streptococcus pneumoniae* antigen by a rapid immunochromatographic assay in urine samples. Chest 2001; 119: 243-249.

45. Murray PR, Washington JA. Microscopic and bacteriologic analysis of expectorated sputum. Mayo Clin Proc 1975; 50: 339-44.

46. NOW® *Streptococcus pneumoniae* antigen test. Product instructions 2003; Rev. 2: 2-80.

47. Bohte R, van Furth R, van den Broek PJ. A etiology of community-acquired pneumonia: a prospective study among adults requiring admission to hospital. Thorax 1995; 50: 543-7.

48. Bella F, Tort J, Morera MA, Espaulella J, Armengol J. Value of bacterial antigen detection in the diagnostic yield of transthoracic needle aspiration in severe community acquired pneumonia. Thorax 1993; 48: 1227-9.

49. Woodhead M. Community-acquired pneumonia in Europe: causative pathogens and resistance patterns. Eur Respir J 2002; Suppl 36: 20s-27s.

50. Sohn JW, Park SC, Choi Y, Woo HJ, et al. Atypical Pathogens as Etiologic Agents in Hospitalized Patients with Community-Acquired Pneumonia in Korea: a prospective multicenter study. J Korean Med Sci 2006; 21: 602-7.

51. Lim WS, Macfarlane JT, Boswell TC, Harrison TG, Rose D, Leinonen M, et al. Study of community acquired pneumonia etiology (SCAPA) in adults admitted to hospital: implications for management guidelines. Thorax 2001; 46: 296-301.

52. Ruiz M, Ewig S, Marcos MA, Martinez JA, Arancibia F, Mensa J, et al. Etiology of community-acquired pneumonia: impact of age, comorbidity, and severity. Am J Respir Crit Care Med 1999; 160: 397-405.

53. Neill AM, Martin IR, Weir R, Anderson R, Chereshsky A, Epton MJ, et al. Community acquired pneumonia: an etiology and usefulness of severity criteria on admission. Thorax 1996; 51: 1010-6.

54. Mandell LA, Bartlett JG, Dowell SF, File TM Jr, Musher DM, Whitney C. Update of practice guidelines for the management of community-acquired pneumonia in immunocompetent adults. Clin Infect Dis 2003; 37: 1405-33.

55. Guchev LA, Yu VL, Sinopalnikov A, Klochkov OI, Koslov RS, Stratchounski LS. Management of nonsevere pneumonia in military trainees with urinary antigen test for Streptococcus pneumoniae: an innovative approach to targeted therapy. Clin Infect Dis 2005; 40: 1608-16.

56. Luna CM, Calmaggi A, Caberloto O, Gentile J, Valentini R, Ciruzzi J, et al. Community-acquired pneumonia. Practice guideline prepared by an inter-society committee. Medicina (Buenos Aires) 2003; 63: 319-43.

57. Geckler RW, Gremillion DH, MacAllister CK, et al. Microscopic and bacteriological comparison of paired sputum and transtracheal aspirates. J Clin Microbiol 1977; 6: 396.

58. Marrie TJ, Durant H, Yates L. Community-acquired pneumonia requiring hospitalization. Rev Infect Dis 1989; 11: 586.

59. Smith PR. What Diagnostic Tests Are Needed for Community-Acquired Pneumonia? Med Clin N Am 2001; 85: 1381-97.

60. Skerrett SJ. Diagnostic testing for community-acquired pneumonia. Clin Chest Med 1999;

20: 531.

61. Corrêa RA, Lopes RM, Oliveira LM, Campos FT, Reis MA, Rocha MO. Study of cases hospitalized for community-acquired pneumonia over a one-year period. J Pneumol 2001; 27: 243-8.

62. Musher DM, Montoya R, Wanahita A. Diagnostic Value of Microscopic Examination of Gram-Stained Sputum and Sputum Cultures in Patients with Bacteremic Pneumococcal Pneumonia. Clin Infect Dis 2004; 39: 165-9.

63. Ewig S, Schlochtermeier M, Goke N, Niederman MS. Applying Sputum as a Diagnostic Tool in Pneumonia: Limited Yeld, Minimal Impact on Treatment Decisions. Chest 2002; 121(5): 1486-92.

64. Huang HH, Zhang Y, Xiu QY, Zhou X, Huang SG, Lu Q, Wang DM, Wang F. Community-acquired pneumonia in Shanghai, China: microbial etiology and implications for empirical therapy in a prospective study of 389 patients. Eur J Clin Microbiol Infect Dis 2006; 25: 369-374.

65. Rosón B, Sabé NF, Carratalà J, Verdaguer R, Dorca J, Manresa F, Gudiol F. Contribution of antigen assay (Binax NOW) to the early diagnosis of pneumococcal pneumonia. Clin Infect Dis 2004; 38: 222-6.

66. Waterer GW, Wunderink RG. The influence of the severity of community-acquired pneumonia on the usefulness of blood cultures. Respir Med 2001; 95: 78-82.

67. Diaz AF, Calvo MA, O'Brien AS, Farias GG, Mardónez JM, Saldias FP. Clinical utility of blood cultures in patients hospitalized for community-acquired pneumonia. Rev Méd Chile 2002; 130: 993-1000.

68. Kollef MH, Shorr A, Tabak YP, Gupta V, Liu LZ, Johannes RS. Epidemiology and Outcomes of Health-care-Associated Pneumonia: results from a large us database of culture-positive pneumonia. Chest 2005; 128: 3854-62.

69. Tleyjeh IM, Tlaygeh HM, Hejal R, Montotori VM, Baddour LM. The Impact of Penicillin Resistance on Short-Term Mortality in Hospitalized Adults with Pneumococcal Pneumonia: a systematic review and meta-analysis. Clin Infect Dis 2006; 42: 778-97.

70. Moine P, Vercken JB, Chevret S, Chastang C, Gajdos P. Severe community-acquired pneumonia. Etiology, epidemiology, and prognosis factors. French Study Group for Community-Acquired Pneumonia in the Intensive Care Unit. Chest 1994; 105: 1487-95.

71. Leroy O, Santre C, Beuscart C, Georges H, Guery B, Jacquier JM, et al. A five-year study of severe community-acquired pneumonia with emphasis on prognosis in patients admitted to an intensive care unit. Intensive Care Med 1995; 21: 24-31.

72. Georges H, Leroy O, Vandenbussche C, Guery B, Alfandari S, Tronchon L, et al. Epidemiological features and prognosis of severe community-acquired pneumococcal pneumonia. Intensive Care Med 1999; 25: 198-206.

73. Rioseco ML, Riquelme RO. Neumococcal bacteremic neumonia in 45 hospitalized immunocompetent adults. Clinical picture and prognostic factors. Ver Méd Chile 2004; 132: 588-594.

74. Metersky ML, Ma A, Bratzler DW, Houck PM. Predicting Bacteremia in Patients with Community-Acquired Pneumonia. Am J Respir Crit Care Med 2004; 169: 342-347.

75. Marcos MA, Gonzalez L, Angrill L, et al. The urinary antigen test for improvement of the diagnosis of Community-acquired pneumonia [abstract]. Am J Respir Crit Care Med 2000; 161: A294.

76. Stralin K, Kaltoft MS, Konradsen HB, Olcén P, Holmberg H. Comparison of two

urinary antigen tests for establishment of pneumococcal etiology of adult community-acquired pneumonia. J Clin Microbiol 2004; 42: 3620-3625.

77. Macfarlane JT, Smith WHR, Morris AH, Rose DH. Comparative radiographic features of community-acquired Legionnaires disease, pneumococcal pneumonia, Mycoplasma pneumonia, and psittacosis. Thorax 1984; 39: 28-33.

78. Tew J, Calenoff L, Brlin BS. Bacterial or nonbacterial pneumonia: accuracy of radiography diagnosis. Radiology 1977; 124: 607-612.

79. Ponka A, Sarna S. Differential diagnosis of viral, mycoplasmal and bacteremic pneumococcal pneumonias on admission to hospital. Eur J Resp Dis 1983; 64: 360-368.

80. Fernandéz MR, Zagolin MB, Ruiz MC, Martinez MA, Diaz JC. Neumonia acquired in the hospitalized community: etiological study. Rev Méd Chile 2003; 131: 498-504.

81. Halm EA, Teirstein AS. Management of Community-Acquired Pneumonia. N Engl J Med 2002; 347: 2039-45.

82. Arnold FW, Ramirez JA, McDonald C, Xia EL. Hospitalization for Community-Acquired Pneumonia: the pneumonia severity index vs clinical judgment. Chest 2003; 124: 121-124.

83. Menéndez R, Torres A, Castro FR, Zalacain R, Aspa J, Villasclaras JJM, Borderias L, et al. Reaching Stability in Community-Acquired Pneumonia: The efectes of the Severity of Disease, Treatment, and the Characteristics of Patients. Clin Infect Dis 2004; 39: 1783-90.

84. Sanyal S, Smith PR, Saha AC, Gupta S, Berkowitz L, Homel P. Initial microbiologic studies did not affect outcome in adults hospitalized with community-acquired pneumonia. Am J Respir Crit Care Med 1999; 160: 346-8.

85. Ewig S, Ruiz M, Mensa J. et al. Severe community-acquired pneumonia: assesment of severity criteria. Am J Respir Crit Care Med 1998; 158: 1102-1108.

86. Chilean Society of Respiratory Diseases and Chilean Society of Infectious Diseases. Management of community-acquired adult neumonia. Summary of the national consensus. Rev Méd Chile 2005; 133: 953-967.

87. Menéndez R, Torres A, Zalacain R, Aspa J, Martin-Villasclaras JJ, et al. Guidelines for the Treatment of Community-acquired Pneumonia: predictors of adherence and outcome. Am J Respir Crit Care Med 2005; 172: 757-762.

88. Musher DM. How Contagious Are Common Respiratory Tract Infections. N Engl J Med 2003; 348: 1256-66.

89. Roux A, Marcos MA, Garcia E, Mensa J, Ewig S, Lode H, Torres A. Viral Community-Acquired Pneumonia in Nonimmunocompromised Adults. Chest 2004; 125: 1343-1351.

90. Diaz AF, Torres CM, Flores LJS, Garcia PC, Saldias FP. Community-acquired neumococcal pneumonia in hospitalized adults. Rev Méd Chile 2003; 131: 505-14.

91. Boersma WG, Lowenberg A, Holloway Y, et al. Pneumococcal capsular antigen detection and pneumococcal serology in patients with community acquired pneumonia. Thorax 1991; 46: 902-906.

92. Rello J, Bodi M, Mariscal D, Navarro M, Diaz E, et al. Microbiological Testing and Outcome of Patients With Severe Community-Acquired Pneumonia. Chest 2003; 123: 174180.

93. Campbell SG, Marrie JT, Anstey R, Dickinson G, et al. The Contribution of Blood Cultures to the Clinical Management of Adult Patients Admitted to the Hospital With Community- Acquired Pneumonia. Chest 2003; 123: 1142-50.

94. Rocha RT, Vital AC, Silva COS, et al. Community-acquired pneumonia in outpatients: epidemiologic, clinical and radiologic aspects of atypical and non-atypical pneumonias. J Pneumol 2000; 26: 5-14.

95. Burke AC. Community-Acquired Pneumonia: diagnostic and therapeutic approach. Med Clin N Am 2001; 85 43-77.

96. Marston BJ, Plouffe JF, File TM, Hackman BA. Incidence of community-acquired pneumonia requiring hospitalization: results of a population-based active surveillance study in ohio. Arch Inter Med 1997; 157: 1709-1718.

97. Gil RD, Undurraga AP, Saldias FP, Jiménez PP, Barros MM, et al. Multicenter study of prognostic factors in adults hospitalized for community-acquired pneumonia. Ver méd Chile 2006; 134: 1357-1366.

98. Marrie JT, Wu L. Factors Influencing In-hospital Mortality in Community-Acquired Pneumonia: a prospective study of patients not initially admitted to the ICU. Chest 2005; 127: 1260-70.

99. Ewig S, Roux A, Bauer T, Garcia E, Mensa J, Niederman M, Torres A. Validation of predictive rules and indices of severity for community acquired pneumonia. Thorax 2004; 59(5): 421-427.

100. Kaplan V, Angus DC, Griffin MF, Clermont G, Watson RS. Hospitalized Community-acquired Pneumonia in the Elderly: age- and sex-related patterns of care and outcome in the United States. Am J Respir Crit Care Med 2002; 165: 766-772.

101. Angus DC, Marrie TJ, Obrosky DS, Clermont G, Dremnizov TT, et al. Severe Community-acquired Pneumonia: use of intensive care services and evaluation of american and british thoracic society diagnostic criteria. Am J Respir Crit Care Med 2002; 166: 717723.

102. Ebell MH. Outpatient vs. Inpatient Treatment of Community-Acquired Pneumonia: using a clinical prediction tool at the point of care will help you choose which course is best for your patient. Family Practice Management april 2006: 41-44.

103. Falguera M, Pifarre R, Martin A, Sheikh A, Moreno A. Etiology and Outcome of Community-Acquired Pneumonia in Patients With Diabetes Mellitus. Chest 2005; 128: 3233-3239.

104. British Thoracic Society. British Thoracic Guidelines for management of community-acquired pneumonia in adults. Thorax 2001; 56 (Suppl 4): 1-64

105. Mandell LA, Marrie TJ, Grossman RF, et al. Canadian guidelines for initial management of community acquired pneumonia: an evidence-based update by the Canadian Infectious Diseases Society and Canadian Thoracic Society. Clin Infect Dis 2000; 31: 383-421.

106. Mandell LA, Niederman MS. The Canadian community-acquired pneumonia consensus group. Antimicrobial treatment of community acquired pneumonia in adults: a conference report. Can J Infect Dis 1993; 4: 25-28.

107. Diaz FA, Labarca JL, Pérez CC, Ruiz MC, Wolf MR. Treatment of community-acquired adult neumonia. Rev Chil Enf Respir 2005; 21: 117-31.

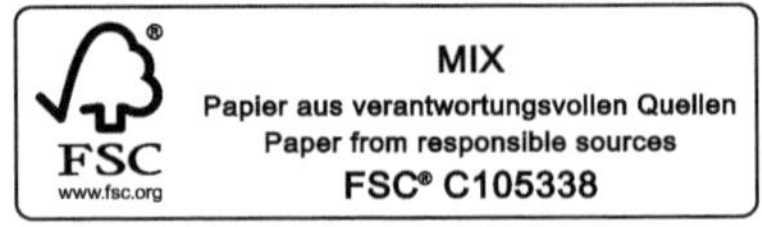

Printed by Books on Demand GmbH, Norderstedt / Germany